Amira El-Houfey
Mohammed Areeshi

Keep the environment clean

Amira El-Houfey
Mohammed Areeshi

Keep the environment clean

LAP LAMBERT Academic Publishing

Impressum / Imprint

Bibliografische Information der Deutschen Nationalbibliothek: Die Deutsche Nationalbibliothek verzeichnet diese Publikation in der Deutschen Nationalbibliografie; detaillierte bibliografische Daten sind im Internet über http://dnb.d-nb.de abrufbar.
Alle in diesem Buch genannten Marken und Produktnamen unterliegen warenzeichen-, marken- oder patentrechtlichem Schutz bzw. sind Warenzeichen oder eingetragene Warenzeichen der jeweiligen Inhaber. Die Wiedergabe von Marken, Produktnamen, Gebrauchsnamen, Handelsnamen, Warenbezeichnungen u.s.w. in diesem Werk berechtigt auch ohne besondere Kennzeichnung nicht zu der Annahme, dass solche Namen im Sinne der Warenzeichen- und Markenschutzgesetzgebung als frei zu betrachten wären und daher von jedermann benutzt werden dürften.

Bibliographic information published by the Deutsche Nationalbibliothek: The Deutsche Nationalbibliothek lists this publication in the Deutsche Nationalbibliografie; detailed bibliographic data are available in the Internet at http://dnb.d-nb.de.
Any brand names and product names mentioned in this book are subject to trademark, brand or patent protection and are trademarks or registered trademarks of their respective holders. The use of brand names, product names, common names, trade names, product descriptions etc. even without a particular marking in this work is in no way to be construed to mean that such names may be regarded as unrestricted in respect of trademark and brand protection legislation and could thus be used by anyone.

Coverbild / Cover image: www.ingimage.com

Verlag / Publisher:
LAP LAMBERT Academic Publishing
ist ein Imprint der / is a trademark of
OmniScriptum GmbH & Co. KG
Heinrich-Böcking-Str. 6-8, 66121 Saarbrücken, Deutschland / Germany
Email: info@lap-publishing.com

Herstellung: siehe letzte Seite /
Printed at: see last page
ISBN: 978-3-659-63809-1

Zugl. / Approved by: Post Doctoral dissertation, Egypt, 2014

Dedication

First and foremost, I feel always indebted to (ALLAH) the kindest and most merciful for all countless gifts have offered us

Pursuing this work has not been easy for him, so we wish to express our sincere appreciation to all members who love and encouraged us much, many thanks to M.s Shimaa A. Abd-Elaa who helped us in writing this work, Prof. Farag M. Moftah and Dr. Soad Sayed Bayomi, who helped us in revising this work. These words are not enough to convey our deep heart feelings:

To our parent'
To husband/ wife

To our daughters/ suns

To all members of our family and close friends

Dr .Amira A. El- Houfey
&
Dr. Mohammed Y Areeshi

List of Abbreviation

Abbreviation	Meaning
CDC	Centers for Disease Control
CHN	Community Health Nurse
DHF	Dengue Hemorrhagic Fever
E-coli	Escherichia-coli
EDHS	Egyptian Demographic and Health Survey
HAV	Hepatitis A Virus
HIV	Human Immune Virus
IG	Immunoglobulin
MOHP	Ministry of Health and Population
MSW	Municipal Solid Waste
NRDC	Natural Resources Defense Council
S. typhi	Salmonella typhi
UNEP	United Nation Environmental Program
WHO	World Health Organization

List of Contents

1-Introduction:

Wastes are considered as one of the most concerning environmental problems that every associated organization has to be aware of environmental problems. All the organizations that are involved with the problem must co-operate and try to solve this crisis together because it is a problem that occurs at every community level ranging from villages to large metropolitans. The problem of wastes seems to become more severe as time passes due to the growth in the country's economics as well as other developments **(Kaewsawang, 2002)**.

Solid wastes from a certain community usually consists of a mixture of wastes and management of household wastes is also a major issue especially in rural areas because wastes collection and disposal systems are virtually not exists. Poor environmental condition causes a large proportion of the global burden of disease. Maintenance of environmental goods and services underpins all aspects of human health and well being **(Min, 2009)**.

Household waste is a movable solid item arising from human activities, that is discarded as useless or unwanted and derived from house and that has no positive value one. Household solid waste is considered controlled wastes and consist of many different things including food, garden waste, paper, card board, glass, metal, plastics and textiles. Agricultural waste is considered not controlled wastes and comprises mainly slurry and farmyard manure with

4

significant quantities of straw, silage effluent and vegetable and cereal residues. Most of this is spread on land **(Fischer and Crowe, 2000).**

Improper disposal of household products can cause a lot of health problem to the people and also to the waste collector. From this problem irritation in nose, eye, gastrointestinal problem, E.g. (diarrhea, dysentery), fatigue, headache, psychological problem and allergies. Over crowded housing may exacerbate problems in managing human waste, which may taint food stuffs and contribute to the spread of communicable disease **(Nies and McEwen, 2012).**

Management of solid waste reduces or eliminates adverse impacts on the environment and human health and supports economic development and improved quality of life. A number of processes are involved in effectively managing waste for a municipality. These include monitoring, collection, transport, processing, recycling and disposal. From this method reduce; recycling, open burning, incineration, dumping and land fill **(United Nations, 2000).**

Due to improper disposal of household products such as toxic insect spray, some household cleaners, partially used paint cans, used auto oil and termite fumigation chemicals causes health dangers. The availability of toxic substances in the home is especially dangerous to young children. Estimate for 2001 in United state are that nearly 40% of toxic agent most commonly ingested by children younger than 6 years of age included cosmetics, cleaning products, topical agent, pesticides, art/ craft/ office supplies and hydrocarbons **(Allender et al., 2010).**

According to Egypt Demographic and Health Survey (EDHS) 2008 total number of disposal of waste in rural area at upper Egypt are 3,865 million tons according to 2008 Estimate **(EL-Zanaty and Way, 2009).** Solid waste constitute a big environmental problem. It is also a source of many health and hygiene problem and causes a lot of diseases to people and scavenger. In rural areas, waste collection and disposal systems are virtually non existent**(Zayani and Riad, 2010).**

Approximately 1.8 million people die worldwide every year from diarheal diseases and malaria. About 88 % of diarrheal diseases and malaria are attributed to poor sanitation and poor hygiene **(Ministry of Public Health and Sanitation, 2011).**

Study has been carry out at Rewa Province at 2006 reported that 60% of households people suffering from waste-related illness such as diarrhea and other gastrointestinal-related illness. Only a small percentage of household's people reported any one suffering from dengue fever **(Padma et al, 2006).**

Household wastes are waste which is generated in the day to day operations of a household. It can include everything from lawn clippings to burn out light bulbs. Many movements designed to get people thinking about environmentally friendly living have focused on household waste as something which can be easily manipulated

6

to make a difference in the environment. Management of household waste is also a major issue and it has been for hundreds of years. When the amount of wastes that are produced and become substantially high which not all the wastes can be properly handled and treated then this would bring about many others problems to the environment **(Naing, 2009).**

Solid waste is the unwanted or useless solid materials generated from combined residential, industrial and commercial activities in a given area. It may be categorized according to its origin (domestic, industrial, commercial, construction or institutional); according to its contents (organic material, glass, metal, plastic paper etc); or according to hazard potential (toxic, non-toxin, flammable, radioactive, infectious etc) **(Jonton, 2006).**

Household solid waste is one of the most difficult sources of solid waste to manage because of its diverse range of composite materials. A substantial portion is made up of garbage, a term for the waste matter that arises from the preparation, and consumption of food and consists of waste food, vegetable peelings and other organic matter. Other components of household solid waste include plastics, paper, glass, textiles, cellophane, metals and some hazardous waste from household products such as paint, garden pesticides, pharmaceuticals, fluorescent tubes, personal care products, batteries containing heavy metals and discarded wood treated with dangerous substances such as anti-fungal and anti-termite chemicals. Also, from wastes found in rural areas animal, bird and agricultural wastes **(Azikiwe et al., 2013).**

Most solid wastes are disposed on the land in open dumps. Disposal of solid waste on the land without careful planning and management can present a danger to the environment and the human health. The environment should be clean and less polluted by all means. This means that waste should be managed at all costs to limit its effects to the environment **(US Environmental Protection Agency, 2006).**

Management of solid waste reduces or eliminates adverse impacts on the environment and human health and supports economic development and improved quality of life. A number of processes are involved in effectively managing waste for a municipality. These include monitoring, collection, transport, processing, recycling and disposal **(Jonton, 2006).**

Methods of waste reduction, waste reuse and recycling are the preferred options when managing waste. There are many environmental benefits that can be derived from the use of these methods. They reduce or prevent green house gas emissions, reduce the release of pollutants, conserve resources, save energy and reduce the demand for waste treatment technology and landfill space. Therefore it is advisable that these methods be adopted and incorporated as part of the waste management plan **(Miller, 2002).**

Community health nurse (CHN) can encourage the positive action described by educating the public, nurse can promote greater sensitivity among citizen to the problems of accumulating waste with its potential health hazards. Public cooperation with organized refuse collection will require a considerable effort by community worker. Nurse encourage client to buy products that can be recycled and discourage use of non recyclable items. CHN must sharing information with people during home visits and make family and home assessment **(Allender et al., 2010).** The primary responsibilities of the CHN are advocacy and education of the client in the home, at work and in the community. Primary prevention is to focus of the educating people about safe solid wastes disposal methods. Nurse make intervention to help in minimizing the potential for illness transmission from insect and rodents that can come in contact with infectious agents and cause spread of disease **(Smith and Maurer, 2000).**

2- Definition of terms and concept:

Terms which will be defined in this study include the following household, wastes, solid waste, household solid wastes, disposal, household waste management, rural and health.

Concept of household waste management:

Household, is defined as a social unit, comprised of people living in the same house, with a head and pooling their incomes together for the management of their dwelling unit. This incomes is pooled together for food, shelter and other social needs and for the general management of the household, including household wastes management **(Jonton, 2006).**

Wastes, generally refers to all unwanted and economically unusable materials that result from human activities, discarded purposefully or accidentally for environment **(Jonton, 2006).**

Solid wastes, are general wastes that are not a liquid or a gas, originating from industrials, household, municipal or agricultural sources**(Miller,2002).**

Household solid wastes, is defined as the day to day rubbish, garbage and other forms of wastes such as kitchen wastes, food packaging, etc...originating from the household **(Van Beukering et al., 2005).**

Household wastes, include ordinary refuse, garbage, swill, rubbish and all forms of refuse from household activities. This household wastes can be in the form of a solid or liquids (**Jonton, 2006).**

Disposal, refers to all activities under taken to get rid of household wastes through sorting, collecting, transporting and disposal in designated locations for treatment, recycling or re-use **(Miller, 2002).**

Health, is defined as a state of complete physical, mental and social well-being and not merely the absence of disease or infirmity **(Jonton, 2006).**

Household waste management, is control of waste material resulting from house and municipal process and effort to minimize waste production **(Nies and McEwen, 2012).**

3-Types of household waste:

Household waste consist of many different things including food, garden waste, paper card board, glass, metal, plastics and textiles. Certain type of waste is defined as hazardous because of inherent characteristics e.g. (toxic, explosive). The three largest waste streams in this category are oils, oily waste, construction and demolition waste, asbestos and wastes from organic chemical process as medication, paints, light bubs, batteries and pesticide containers **(Fischer and Crowe, 2000).**

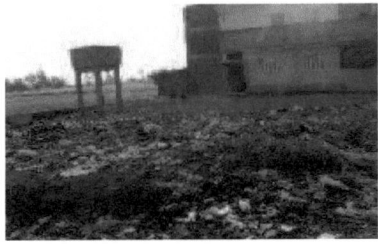 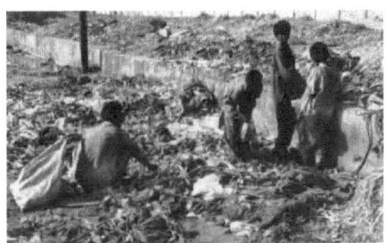

Figure (1): Open dumpsites - 'Haven for scavengers'

There are five board categories of domestic wastes:-

1- Biodegradable waste: as food and kitchen waste, green waste, paper.

2- Recyclable material: as paper, glass, cans, metals, certain plastics...etc.

3- Inert waste: as construction and demolition waste, dirt, rocks and debris.

4- Composite waste: as waste clothing, tetra paks, waste plastics such as toys.

5- Hazardous waste (also, called "Household Hazardous Waste") and toxic waste: as medication, electronic-waste, paints, chemicals, light bulbs, fluorescent tubes, spray cans, pesticide containers, batteries and shoe polish **(Pheby et al., 2002).**

4- Types of waste in rural areas:

In rural areas people look after the animal in their home with its risk on human health. In addition to dust, the offensive odors from cattle, poultry and swine operations can be overwhelming. Individuals manage animal waste by sweeping it into a rubbish heap, dumping it in the nearby bush or washing it directly into rivers. It is commonly left in the open and during rainy weather organic matter and bacteria enter the water system .While many traditional crop and livestock operations use manure as a fertilizer, letting animals roam on land after harvest to build up organic matter **(Natural Resources Defence Council, 2006).**

Raw manure from cattle and poultry can contain up to 100 million fecal coliform bacteria per gram, as well as ammonia, phosphorus and other nutrients and microbes that can contaminate soil and water in high concentration. Escherichia- coli (E.coli) bacteria have been found in the manure of a quarter of the beef cattle on large feedlots **(Wallinga, 2004).**

In addition to, manure from cattle and poultry there are agricultural waste it is considered not controlled and comprises mainly slurry and farmyard manure with significant quantities of straw, silage effluent and vegetable and cereal residues. Most of this is spread on land **(Fischer and Crowe, 2000).**

Crops residuals used to be stored by farmers on top of their roofs to be used as a source of fuel when burned. However, the increasing spread of propane / butane gas fired ovens and stoves resulted in decreasing the use of waste as a fuel. Moreover, new regulations were introduced by the Ministry of Agriculture to ban the storage of agricultural waste as a measure to fight pests and diseases, and to prevent hazardous fires. Due to the lack of resources, farmers prefer to dispose off the undesired, no storable waste by illegal means such as burning or random dumping. This reduced the utilization rate of agricultural waste from 100% to 40% **(Zayani and Riad, 2010).**

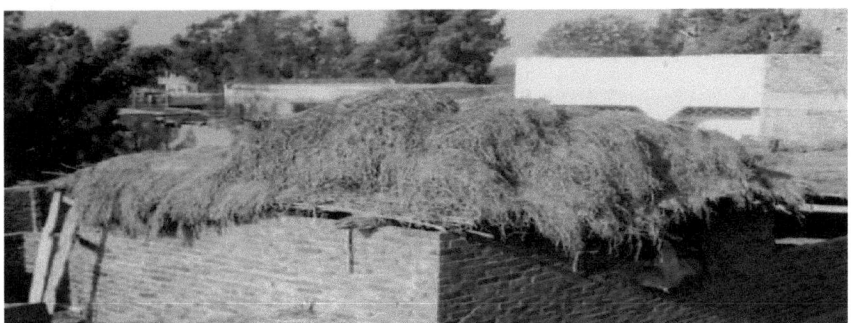

Figure (2): Using straw in rural areas give the chance to rats and insects spread

Farm households in rural communities generate solid organic wastes such as manure, tree trimmings, grass clippings and crop

13

residues. Organic wastes can amount up to 80 percent of the total solid wastes generated in any farm household. Also, livestock generate large amounts of wastes. Manure production can amount up to 5.27 kg/day/1000 kg live weight, on a wet weight basis **(Mohee, 2001).**

The organic wastes, especially manure generated by animals, if improperly managed or left untreated can result in significant degradation of soil, water and air quality. Stagnant wastes provide a medium in which flies breed and diseases are transmitted. Uncontrolled decomposition of organic wastes produces odorous gases as well as ammonia volatilization, leading to acid rain. Odors generated at production and manure storage facilities are the most frequent source of complaints against animal producers. Because of the intensification of animal production on a small area of land, there are increasing concerns about:
• Water quality resulting from higher nitrogen and phosphorous loadings.
• Pathogens and antimicrobial compounds in the manure.
• Foul odors and air quality from ammonia, methane and nitrous oxide emissions.
• Soil quality because of potassium and phosphorous loading **(Mohee, 2001).**

Farmers and gardeners have long recognized the importance of replacing nutrients and organic matter that are depleted under continuous cropping. They have been applying directly raw or partially treated wastes to the fields. Potential problems related to nutrient management, such as nutrient overloading, nutrient losses and high salt levels have been associated with the direct application of manure. In addition, manure has to be stored to enable it to be incorporated in the soil at scheduled times and some farmers may not have available cropland to effectively incorporate the volumes generated day after day. Also, some farmers may not have an adequate area of land to use in a sustainable manner all the nutrients in manure (**Mohee, 2001).**

Organic wastes can be converted easily to a resource for farm households through composting. Composting agricultural and other types of wastes can be a useful process for recycling nutrients and maintaining or restoring levels of organic matter in the soil. Composting can be an attractive, low-cost technology for farmers. Because composted waste is treated, it is more stable than untreated or partially treated wastes **(Solano et al., 2001).**

The composting fundamentals for individual on-farm projects are similar to rural community composting projects. Farmers generating low amounts of wastes can join together to compost larger amounts of wastes in bigger community facilities creating a more efficient way of generating income **(Mohee, 2001).**

People in rural community have some bad habits in hygiene. They look after the animal in their home and they dispose the waste of this animal by bad method for example they using cattle disposal in the bio stove and this methods pollute the rural house, look after the cultivate poultry on the roofs without cleaning. This is a bad

15

aspect in the cities or rural areas, they saving the cattle disposal on the house roof may pollute the environment and spread the harmful insects and using straw in rural areas give the chance to rats and insects spread and all this bad habits make the people in rural community has high chance of spread of disease **(Nour Eldeein, 2011).**

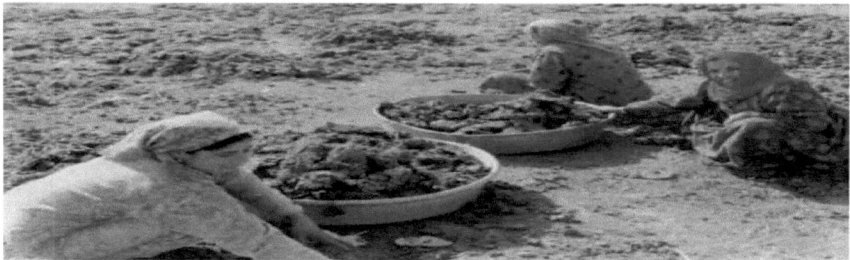

Figure (3): Using cattle manure in the bio stove is pollute the rural house

5- Methods of household solid waste management:-

Waste management mean control of waste material resulting from municipal process, house or human consumption and effort to minimize waste production by a lot of method. The management of solid waste is today one of the important obligatory functions of the local government areas in the entire country. However, this vary important and essential service had in the past gulped a lot of money out of the local authorities, that the state government's intervention became necessary. The reason is not far fetched, the Local Government Areas were not properly, technically and financially equipped to perform this statutory function well. The banes of the problem include but not limited to lack of financial resources, weak institutional and legal frame work. Others are in appropriate choice of technology, in adequate collection and transportation systems as well as unsafe final disposal options **(Longe and Khinde, 2005).**

Even though the fundamental objectives of any solid waste management programme are to minimize environmental pollution, these goals become unachievable in the absence of sustained funding, affordable local technological option and lack of participatory approach to integrated solid waste management **(Longe and Williums, 2006).**

Household solid waste management encompasses the full range of management activities from household waste streams from the point of generating the waste to the point of disposal. These activities largely focus on resources recovery which includes all the activity entailed in waste segregation, collection and processing, which are carried out taking into consideration economic viability of the material that is being recovered, e.g. for re-use and recycling **(Language and Van Blerk, 2000).**

The major methods of waste management are:-

- Recycling- the recovery of materials from products after they have been used by consumers.
- Composting- an aerobic, biological process of degradation of biodegradable organic matter.
- Incineration- a process of combustion designed to recover energy and reduce the volume of waste going to disposal.
- Land fill- the deposition of waste in a specially designated area, which in modern sites consist of a pre-constructed 'cell' lined with an

impermeable layer (man-made or natural) and with controls to minimize emissions.

• Sewage treatment- a process of treating raw sewage to produce a non-toxic liquid effluent which is discharged to rivers and a semi-solid sludge, which is used as a soil amendment on land, incinerated or disposed of in land fill **(Pheby et al., 2002).**

Reuse and recycling:

Reuse and recycling are conceptualized as processes which provide an opportunity to capture some of the values from waste. Of the two concepts, reuse is a simpler technique involving the re-utilization of material in its end use form without the necessity of further value addition or reprocessing. Recycling on the other hand, involves processing waste through conversion of parts or all of the waste into other useful material or to recover the original raw matter. While recycling and reuse provide an opportunity to regain residual value of waste material or transform waste into usable raw materials, the resource requirements (energy, human resources...etc) may some times be vary great. These resource requirements can be greatly reduced through waste prevention, collection and treatment **(Jonton, 2006).**

Waste prevention, collection and treatment:

Waste prevention is defined as all the activities and efforts of individuals and groups of individuals undertaken to minimize the volume of domestic waste generated or generate waste in a form that facilitates easy collection, treatment and recycling. The collection of waste and its recovery from different waste generating points is carried out by many agents such as formal and informal, which may represent a variety of organization structure and relationships **(UNEP, 2002).**

In developing countries, solid waste management come under the auspices of municipal bodies, which are the formal bodies responsible for the collection, removal and disposal of garbage from public specific areas of action on improving the efficiency of waste management, as summarized in United Nation Environmental Programme (UNEP) at 2002 include:-

- Waste prevention, minimization and waste detoxification.
- Waste collection, transfer, transport and storage.
- Waste treatment, including waste disposal.

In the developed countries, different technologies may be available for waste treatment and recycling generally, four main groups of waste treatment methods exists these include:-

1. Biological treatment:

This generally entails the transformation of waste into organic matter via composting and aerobic transformation this treated waste then becomes useful nutrients in agricultural production at home or on the farms.

2. Incineration:

Entails burning waste materials or substances with or without recovering some or all of the energy for reuse.

3. Land fill:

This is a controlled method in developed countries, where waste is stored and biodegradable components disposed on controlled landfill sites.

4. Dumping:

Apart from these controlled methods. Which are mostly prevalent in the developed and developing countries, uncontrolled methods can often not be avoided especially in the developing world. In large parts of Africa, for instance, solid waste is still dumped in the open air, in the ocean, or by burning it on site. Such ways of disposal have irreversible and potentially harmful effects on both human health and the environment. These clearly not methods that belong to sustainable waste managements. It is alarming to note from a recent assessment that, such disposal methods are frequently employed in an estimated 175 sovereign nations and territories **(UNEP, 2002).**

Dumping and burning are the most common solid waste disposal methods. Dumping is a problematic because garbage dumps provide perfect conditions for breeding of rats, flies and other disease-carrying organisms and may potentially be a source of water contamination from run off. Dumps also are eyesores that take up valuable land resources. Burning, although it reduces the volume of garbage, produce noxious odors and pollutes the air. Sanitary landfills have generally replaced dumps as a more effective way to dispose of refuse by burning it. With proper handling, including covering and daily sealing (to prevent insect and rodent breeding), this method has proven satisfactory for handling of solid waste **(Spradley and Allender, 2008).**

6- Vector-borne diseases:

"Vector-borne disease" is the term commonly used to describe an illness caused by infectious microbe that is transmitted by a blood-sucking arthropod from an infected vertebrate (e.g., bird, rodent, deer or human) to susceptible person. A vector-borne disease is one in which the pathogenic microorganism is transmitted from an infected individual to another individual by an arthropod or other agent, sometimes with other animals serving as intermediary hosts. Nearly half of the world's population is infected by vector-borne diseases, resulting in high morbidity and mortality. The distribution of the incidence of vector-borne diseases is grossly disproportionate, with the overwhelming impact in developing countries located in tropical and subtropical areas **(Sachs and Malaney, 2002).**

All household waste cause breeding of insects and rodents living in their environment. The most common vectors are mosquitoes, flies, ticks, roaches, fleas, rats, mice, ground squirrels, snakes and scorpion. All of these agents can serve as reservoirs for germs that they then transmit through physical contact with humans or by contaminating human food stuffs or water **(Allender et al., 2010).**

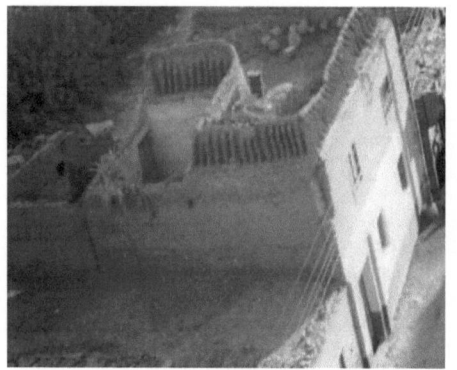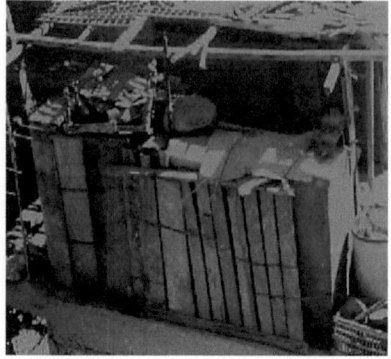

Figure (4): Cultivate poultry on the roofs without cleaning is a bad aspect in rural areas, pollute the environment and spread the harmful insects

All human communities are affected by the insects and rodents living in their environment. Not only are these creatures a nuisance in peoples homes, but they may cause economic damage and create serious health hazards as well. On the least dangerous level they serve as annoying pests that may cause irritation, such as mosquito or fly bites and discomfort, such as infestations of bedbugs or lice. They can also pose a direct threat to health through such things attacks by diseased rats or squirrels. They can consume and in tern contaminate food, but by far the most serious health hazard that they impose is through their role as vectors which are nonhuman carriers of disease organisms that can transmit these organisms directly to humans.

The most common vectors are remembered in the last paragraph. The next table summarizes some of the diseases spread by vectors. Cases of vector-spread diseases range from the fourteenth-century bubonic plague epidemic spread by rat fleas, which killed a quarter of the European population, to the continuing problem of mosquito-spread malaria in no industrialized nations **(Nies and McEwen, 2012).**

Table (I): Some insect vectors and diseases transmitted by insect:-

Pathogen	Disease	Vector
Mosquitoes Anopheles sp Culex sp. Culex sp. Aedes aegypti Aedes aegypti	Malaria Filariasis Encephalitis Yellow fever Dengue	Plasmodium sp. (protozoa) Wucheraria bancrofti ana malayi (nematodes) Arbovirus Arbovirus Arbovirus
Biting Flies Deerfly Black fly Tsetse fly Sand fly	Filariasis River blindness Sleeping sickness Kala-azar Tropical ulcer Cutaneous leishmaniasis Espundia Phlebotomus fever	Loa loa (nematode) Onchocerca volvulus (nematode) Trypanoosoma gambiense and rhodesiense (protozoa) Leshmania donovani Leishmania tropica Leishmania mexicana Leishmania braziliense (protozoa) Arbovirus
Other **Insects** Gnats Rat flea Body Louse Tick Tick Mite	Filariasis Plague Murine typhus Epidemic typhus Trench fever Rocky Mountain spotted fever Colorado tick fever Riskettsialpox	Mansonella ozzardi (nematode) Yersinia pestis (bacteria) Rickettsia mooseri Rickettsia prowazekii Rickettsia Quintana Rickettsia rickettsia Arbovirus Tickettsia akari

Cited from **(Spradly and Allender, 2008).**

The transmission of diseases from vector depends upon the attributes and requirements of at least three different living organisms: the pathologic agent, a virus, protozoa, bacteria, worm; the vectors, which are commonly arthropods such as ticks or mosquitoes; and the human host. In addition, intermediary hosts such as domesticated or wild animals often serve as a reservoir for the pathogen until susceptible human populations are exposed **(Sachs and Malaney, 2002).**

The most deadly vector borne disease, malaria, kills over 1.2 million people annually, mostly African children under the age of five. Dengue fever, together with associated Dengue Hemorrhagic Fever (DHF), is the world's fastest growing vector borne disease. Poorly designed irrigation and water systems, inadequate housing, poor waste disposal and water storage, deforestation and loss of biodiversity, all may be contributing factors to the most common vector-borne diseases including malaria, dengue and leishmaniasis **(Duane, 1998).**

Control measures for vector-borne diseases are important because most are zoonoses that are maintained in nature in cycles involving wild animals and are not amenable to eradication. Control measures can be targeted at several different aspects of the life cycle of vector-borne diseases. Vaccinations for animal and human populations are aimed at preventing the proliferation of pathogen and pesticides reduce or eliminate the vectors. Therefore, control methods generally focus on targeting the arthropod vector. These include undertaking personal protective measures by establishing physical barriers such as house screens and bed nets; wearing appropriate clothing (boots, apparel that overlap the upper garments, head nets, etc.); and using insect repellents. Environmental modification to eliminate specific breeding areas or chemical biological control measures to kill arthropod larvae or adults may be undertaken **(Goddard, 2000)**.

7- Risks and problems associated with solid wastes:

If solid wastes are not managed properly, there are many negative impacts that may result. Some of the most important are mentioned by **(Tadesse, 2004)** in the following list. The relative importance of each depends very much on local conditions.

• Uncollected wastes often end up in drains, causing blockages which result in flooding and unsanitary conditions.

• Flies breed in some constituents of solid wastes, and flies are very effective vectors that spread disease.

• Mosquitoes breed in blocked drains and in rainwater that is retained in discarded cans, tires and other objects. Mosquitoes spread disease, including malaria and dengue.

• Rats find shelter and food in waste dumps. Rats consume and spoil food, spread disease, damage electrical cables and other materials and inflict unpleasant bites.

• The open burning of waste causes air pollution, the products of combustion include dioxins which are particularly hazardous.

• Aerosols and dusts can spread fungi and pathogens from uncollected and decomposing wastes.

• Uncollected waste degrades the rural environment, discouraging efforts to keep streets and open spaces in a clean and attractive condition. Solid waste management is a clear indicator of the effectiveness of a municipal administration - if the provision of this service is inadequate large numbers of citizens are aware of it. Plastic bags are a particular aesthetic nuisance and they cause the death of grazing animals which eat them.

- Waste collection workers face particular occupational hazards, including strains from lifting, injuries from sharp objects and traffic accidents.
- Dumps of waste and abandoned vehicles block streets and other access ways.
- Dangerous items (such as broken glass, razor blades, hypodermic needles, aerosol cans and potentially explosive containers and chemicals from industries) may pose risks of injury or poisoning, particularly to children and people who sort through the waste.
- Heavy refuse collection trucks can cause significant damage to the surfaces of roads that were not designed for such weights.
- Waste items that are recycled without being cleaned effectively or sterilized can transmit infection to later users. (Examples are bottles and medical supplies).
- Polluted water (leachate) flowing from waste dumps and disposal sites can cause serious pollution of water supplies. Chemical wastes (especially persistent organics) may be fatal or have serious effects if ingested, inhaled or touched and can cause widespread pollution of water supplies.
- Large quantities of waste that have not been placed according to

good engineering practice can slip and collapse, burying and killing people.

• Waste that is treated or disposed of in unsatisfactory ways can cause a severe aesthetic nuisance in terms of smell and appearance.

• Liquids and fumes, escaping from deposits of chemical wastes (perhaps formed as a result of chemical reactions between components in the wastes), can have fatal or other serious effects.

• Landfill gas (which is produced by the decomposition of wastes) can be explosive if it is allowed to accumulate in confined spaces (such as the cellars of buildings).

• Methane (one of the main components of landfill gas) is much more effective than carbon dioxide as a greenhouse gas, leading to climate change.

• Fires on disposal sites can cause major air pollution, causing illness and reducing visibility, making disposal sites dangerously unstable, causing explosions of cans, and possibly spreading to adjacent property. Former disposal sites provide very poor foundation support for large buildings, so buildings constructed on former sites are prone to collapse.

8- Effect of waste accumulation on individual health:

Improper disposal of household products can cause a lot of health problem to the people and also to the waste collector. From this problem irritation in nose, eye, gastrointestinal problem, E.g. (diarrhea, dysentery), fatigue, Headache, psychological problem and allergies. Over crowded housing may exacerbate problems in managing human waste, which may taint food stuffs and contribute to the spread of communicable disease **(Nies and McEwen, 2012).**

Poor waste handling practices and inadequate provision of solid waste management facilities in rural areas of developing countries results in indiscriminate disposal and unsanitary environments that pose a threat to the health of residents. Improper handling, storage and disposal of wastes are major causes of environmental pollution, which provides breeding grounds for pathogenic organisms and encourages the spread of infectious diseases. The presence of houseflies in the kitchen during cooking correlated with the incidence of childhood diarrhea. In addition, an association was found between waste burning and the incidence of respiratory health symptoms among adults and children **(Owaduge, 2010).**

Although household refuse does not usually contain such large amount of germs as excreta, it can cause a risk to public health by attracting flies, mosquitoes and rats and allowing them to breed. This may encourage the spread of diarrheal diseases as well as diseases like dengue fever, yellow fever, bancroftian filariasis, bubonic plague, dermatitis and skin diseases. Also, some infectious diseases as bacteria and viruses, leptospirosis, toxocariasis, salmonellosis and tetanus…..etc. So, refuse must always be stored in a container with a tight fitting lid. The container should be emptied regularly and not allowed to over flow. When the refuse container is emptied it should be washed with soap and water or cleaned with dry earth or sand **(United Nation, 2000).**

Due to improper disposal of household products such as toxic insect spray, some household cleaners, partially used paint cans, used auto oil and termite fumigation chemicals causes health dangers. The availability of toxic substances in the home is especially dangerous to young children. Estimate for 2001 are that nearly 40% of toxic agent most commonly ingested by children younger than 6 years of age included cosmetics, cleaning products, topical agent, pesticides, art/ craft/ office supplies and hydrocarbons **(Allender et al., 2010).**

The common diseases that result from accumulation of household waste in rural community:-
a) Gastrointestinal diseases:
1) Diarrhea:
Diarrhea is the condition of having frequent loose or liquid bowel movements. Acute diarrhea is a common cause of death in developing countries and the second most common cause of infant deaths world wide. The loss of fluids through diarrhea can cause severe dehydration which is one cause of death in diarrhea sufferers. Along with water, sufferers also lose dangerous amounts of important salts, electrolytes and other nutrients. Acute diarrhea is usually related to bacterial, viral or parasitic infection. Chronic diarrhea is usually related to functional disorders such as irritable bowel syndrome or inflammatory bowel disease **(Wangen, 2006).**

Diarrhea commonly results from gastroenteritis caused by Bacterial infection, several types of bacteria consumed through contaminated food or water can cause diarrhea. Viral infections: Many viruses cause diarrhea, including rotavirus, Norwalk virus,

29

cytomegalovirus, herpes simplex virus and viral hepatitis. Food intolerances: some people are unable to digest food components such as artificial sweeteners and lactose the sugar found in milk **(Greenberg and Estes, 2009).**

Diarrhea may be accompanied by cramping, abdominal pain, bloating, nausea or an urgent need to use the bathroom. Depending on the cause, a person may have a fever or bloody stools **(Wangen, 2006).**

Treatment: In many cases of diarrhea, replacing lost fluid and salts is the only treatment needed. This is usually by mouth-oral rehydration therapy or in very severe cases, intravenously. Medicines such as lopermide (imodium), bismuth subsalicylate (as found in pepto bismol and Kaopectate) may be beneficial, however they may be contraindicated in certain situations. Prescribed medications sometimes contain pain-killers, such as morphine or codeine to counter the cramps that can accompany diarrhea **(Schiller, 2007).**

Nursing care of people suffer from diarrhea, monitoring fluid, electrolyte by recording intake and output: close mentoring of specific gravity and encourage patient to take adequate amount of fluid: facilitating home health maintenance by specific instruction to patient about hand washing before and after preparation of diet: the patient should be know signs of dehydration : liquids should be at home temperature because cold liquids may increase bowel motility: body temperature control, preventing and treating perineal excoriation **(Marilyn and David, 2007).**

2) Dysentery:

Dysentery is an inflammatory disorder of the intestine, especially of the colon, that results in severe diarrhea containing mucus and/ or blood in the feces. If left untreated, dysentery can be fatal. Acute amebic dysentery causes a sudden high temperature of (40 to 40.6 C°) accompanied by chills and abdominal cramping: profuse, bloody, mucoid diarrhea with tenesmus: and diffuse abdominal tenderness due to extensive rectosigmoid ulcers. Chronic amebic dysentery produces intermittent diarrhea that lasts for 1 to 4 weeks and recurs several times a year. Such diarrhea produces 4 to 8 or (in severe diarrhea, up to 18) foul-smelling mucus and blood tinged stools daily in a patient with a mild fever, vague abdominal cramps, possible weight loss. Symptoms of dysentery include frequent passage of feces, weight loss, anemia, indigestion, blood in stool and dehydration **(Mitchell, 2002).**

Dysentery is usually caused by a bacterial or protozoan infection or infestation of parasitic worms, but can also be caused by a chemical irritant or viral infection. The two most common causes are infection with a bacillus of the shigella group and infestation by an amoeba, Entamobea histolytica. When caused by a bacillus it is called bacillary dysentery and when caused by an amoeba it is called amoebic dysentery. Complications possibly associated with amebic dysentery include infection spreading to the part of the body, dehydration, liver infection, liver abscess and brain abscess **(Navaneethan and Giannella, 2008).**

Methods of prevention of amebic dysentery mentioned in various sources include: avoid contaminated food, keep food away from flies and avoid contaminated water and wash hand before and after of eat **(Gonzales et al., 2009).**

Therapeutic and nursing care management: Dysentery is initially managed by maintaining fluid intake using oral rehydration therapy. If this treatment can not be adequately maintained due to vomiting or the profuseness of diarrhea, hospital admission may be required for intravenous fluid replacement. Ideally, no antimicrobial therapy should be administered until microbiological microscopy and culture studies have established the specific infection involved. When laboratory services are not available, it may be necessary to administer a combination of drugs, including an amoebicidal drug to kill the parasite and an antibiotic to treat any associated bacterial infection **(Mitchell, 2002).**

3) Typhoid fever:

Typhoid fever is a potentially life-threatening illness that is caused by the bacteria Salmonella typhi (S. typhi). Persons with typhoid fever carry the bacteria in their bloodstream and intestinal tract and can spread the infection directly to other people by contaminating food or water. Anyone can get typhoid fever if they drink water or eat food contaminated with the S. typhi bacteria. Travelers visiting developing countries are at greatest risk for getting typhoid fever. Typhoid fever is still common in the developing world, where it affects about 12.5 million persons each year. Only about 400 cases occur each year in the United State **(WHO, 2005).**

WHO (2005) mentioned the sign and symptom of typhoid fever are elevate body temperature up to 40°, gastrointestinal symptom as (diarrhea, constipation, stomach pain) , headache, malaise, non productive cough, slow heart fever and anorexia.

Causes of typhoid fever are you can get typhoid fever by eating or drinking contaminated food or water. Food or water can be contaminated by a food handler with S. typhi, or may be contaminated if sewage accidentally gets into the food or water. Some infected persons may not show any symptoms of typhoid fever but can shed the S. typhi bacteria in their feces for many years. These persons are called typhoid fever "carriers". S. typhi is only found in humans **(WHO, 2005).**

Treatment of typhoid fever Typhoid fever is treated with antibiotics. A person will usually recover in 2-3 days with prompt antibiotic treatment. People that do not get prompt medical treatment may continue to have a fever for weeks or months, and as many as 20% may die from complications of the infection **(WHO, 2005).**

WHO (2005) mentioned some steps for prevention of typhoid fever such as:-
a) Get vaccinated against typhoid fever. Both injectable and oral vaccines are available. Visit a doctor or travel clinic to discuss your vaccination options. Vaccines are not 100% effective, so it is important to take the additional measures listed to prevent typhoid fever.

b) Use careful selection of food and drink while you are in a developing country. This will also help protect you from other illnesses such as cholera, dysentery and hepatitis A.

c) Only use clean water. Buy it bottled or make sure it has been brought to a rolling boil for at least one minute before you drink it. Bottled carbonated water is safer than uncarbonated water.

d) Ask for drinks without ice unless the ice is made from bottled or boiled water.

e) Only eat foods that have been thoroughly cooked.

f) Avoid raw vegetables and fruits that cannot be peeled.

g) When you eat raw fruits or vegetables that can be peeled, wash your hands with soap, then peel them yourself. Do not eat the peelings.

h) Avoid foods and beverages from street vendors. Many travelers get sick from food bought from street vendors.

4) Hepatitis A virus:

Hepatitis is a general term meaning inflammation of the liver and can be caused by a variety of different viruses such as hepatitis A, B, C, D and E. Since the development of jaundice is a characteristic feature of liver disease, a correct diagnosis can only be made by testing patients' sera for the presence of specific antiviral antibodies **(WHO, 2000).**

Hepatitis A is caused by infection with the hepatitis A virus (HAV), a no enveloped and positive stranded Ribonucleic Acid (RNA) virus, first identified by electron microscopy in 1973, classified within the genus hepatovirus of the picornavirus family.

The virus interferes with the liver's functions while replicating in hepatocytes. The individual's immune system is then activated to produce a specific reaction to combat and possibly eradicate the infectious agent. As a consequence of pathological damage, the liver becomes inflamed **(WHO, 2000).**

HAV is transmitted from person-to-person via the faecal-oral route. As (HAV) is abundantly excreted in faeces and can survive in the environment for prolonged periods of time, it is typically acquired by ingestion of faeces-contaminated food or water. Direct person-to-person spread is common under poor hygienic conditions occasionally, it is also acquired through sexual contact (anal-oral) and blood transfusions. People are susceptible to it are not vaccinated against hepatitis A, are at risk of infection. The risk factors for (HAV) infection are related to resistance of it to the environment, poor sanitation in large areas of the world, and abundant (HAV) shedding in faeces. In areas where this virus is highly endemic, the majority of (HAV) infections occur during early childhood **(WHO, 2000).**

Prevention of the disease, the majority of (HAV) infections are spread by the faecal - oral route so, good personal hygiene, high quality standards for public water supplies and proper disposal of sanitary waste have resulted in a low prevalence of (HAV) infections in many well developed societies. Within households, good personal hygiene, including frequent and proper hand washing after bowel movement and before food preparation, are important measures to reduce the risk of transmission from infected individuals before and after their clinical disease becomes apparent. For pre exposure protection, the use of hepatitis A vaccines instead of immunoglobulin (IG) is now highly recommended. Immunization should be a priority for persons at increased risk of acquiring hepatitis A. For post exposure prophylaxis of non-vaccinated people, the passive administration of (IG) can modify the symptoms of infection, provided it is given within 2 weeks of exposure. No special precautions are demanded for vaccinated persons. Universal immunization would successfully control hepatitis A, although at present, high costs and limited availability of vaccines preclude such a recommendation. Eradication, however, can only be achieved through universal vaccination policies as long as (HAV) is not endemic in primates **(WHO, 2000).**

Treatment of (HAV) as no specific treatment exists for hepatitis A, prevention is the most effective approach against the disease. Therapy should be supportive and aimed at maintaining adequate nutritional balance (1 g/kg protein, 30-35 cal/kg). There is no good evidence that restriction of fats has any beneficial effect on the course of the disease. Eggs, milk and butter may actually help provide a correct caloric intake. Alcoholic beverages should not be consumed during acute hepatitis because of the direct hepatotoxic effect of alcohol. On the other hand, a modest consumption of alcohol during convalescence does not seem to be harmful. Hospitalization is usually not required **(WHO, 2000).**

5) Cholera:

Cholera is an acute enteric infection caused by the ingestion of bacterium Vibrio cholerae present in faecally contaminated water or food. Primarily linked to insufficient access to safe water and proper sanitation. Cholera is characterized in its most severe form by a sudden onset of acute watery diarrhea that can lead to death by severe dehydration. The extremely short incubation period - two hours to five days -enhances the potentially explosive pattern of outbreaks, as the number of cases can rise very quickly. About 75% of people infected with cholera do not develop any symptoms. However, the pathogens stay in their faeces for 7 to 14 days and are shed back into the environment, possibly infecting other individuals. Cholera is an extremely virulent disease that affects both children and adults. Unlike other diarrheal diseases, it can kill healthy adults within hours. Individuals with lower immunity, such as malnourished children or people living with Human immune virus (HIV), are at greater risk of death if infected by cholera **(WHO, 2007).**

WHO (2007) put some measures for the prevention of cholera mostly consist of providing clean water and proper sanitation to populations who do not yet have access to basic services. Health education and good food hygiene are equally important. Communities should be reminded of basic hygienic behaviors, including the necessity of systematic hand-washing with soap after defecation and before handing food or eating, as well as safe preparation and conservation of food. Appropriate media, such as radio, television or newspapers should be involved in disseminating health education messages. Community and religious leaders should also be associated to social mobilization campaigns.

Control of disease among people developing symptoms, 80% of episodes is of mild or moderate severity. The remaining 10%-20% of cases develop severe watery diarrhea with signs of dehydration. Once an outbreak is detected, the usual intervention strategy aims to reduce mortality - ideally below 1% - by ensuring access to treatment and controlling the spread of disease. To achieve this, all partners involved should be properly coordinated and those in charge of water and sanitation must be included in the response strategy. Recommended control methods, including standardized case management, have proven effective in reducing the case-fatality rate. The main tools for cholera control are:

• Proper and timely case management in cholera treatment centres;

• Specific training for proper case management, including avoidance of nosocomial infections;

• Sufficient pre-positioned medical supplies for case management (e.g. diarrhoeal disease kits);

• Improved access to water, effective sanitation, proper waste management and vector control;

• Enhanced hygiene and food safety practices;

• Improved communication and public information **(WHO, 2007).**

b) Eye diseases:

Eye diseases generally occurs in response to viral or bacterial infection, allergies, environmental irritant, surgery or trauma. While most cases of conjunctivitis are not too serious it is important to control the severity of the inflammation as well as the duration to be sure to avoid any scarring and permanent damage **(Mahmoud, 2010).**

There are many different types of eye diseases depending on what area of the eye becomes inflamed, each condition differing in its symptoms and severity: **conjunctivitis**, commonly known as pinkeye, conjunctivitis is an inflammation of the conjunctiva which is the clear membrane that covers the outermost layer of the eye and the inner surface of the eyelids. Many causes are associated with this condition including bacterial and viral infections, allergies and eye irritant. **Episcleritis**, an inflammatory condition of the episclera which is the connective tissue between the conjunctiva and sclera. The cause of episcleritis is uncertain **(Caroline, 2008).**

Blepharitis, an inflammation of the eyelids, often as the result of poor hygiene, chronically dry eyes or oily skin. **Keratitis**, an inflammation of the cornea region of the eye. This is often caused by bacterial or fungal infections and is increasingly prevalent in those with poor contact lens hygiene. **Verities**, an inflammation of the eyeball which is generally considered to be one of the more serious forms of eye inflammation. There are also a number of types of vitas depending on what area of the eye ball is infected and these may include: Iritis, Cyclitis, Retinitis and Choroiditis. **Scleritis**, an inflammation of the sclera or white of the eye **(Caroline, 2008).**

Causes of eye diseases: contact lens use may cause inflammation or infection, especially if hygienic measures are not taken. Hands should be washed before any contact with eye. Over use of prescription and over the counter eye drops. Deficiency of vitamin "A" may make more susceptible to eye infections and other eye problems. Allergies are a fairly common cause of conjunctivitis and cause persistent eye irritation. Allergic rhinitis triggered by pollen, seasonal changes, house dust-mites, molds or pets can often result in itchy and inflamed eyes **(Marshall, 2005).**

Some illnesses such as measles, herpes and diabetes may cause eye diseases. Sometimes foreign matter or foreign substances such as dust, grit or plant-sap get trapped under the eyelid causing inflammation and discomfort. Other causes of conjunctivitis include the use of certain eye cosmetics and cosmetics that have exceeded their expiry date, surgery, trauma or injury to the eye, inflammation conditions such as lupus, arthritis and irritable bowel syndrome and viral and bacterial infections **(Marshall, 2005).**

Therapeutic and nursing care management: medical treatment ranges form antibiotic eye lotions and drops, to over the counter solutions, antihistamine tablets and corticosteroids depending on cause and type of eye inflammation. It is important to make sure you know all the side effects of any medication you may be considering as sometimes the medical treatment causes more complications than the actual eye inflammation. The nurse learns the patient how to make a warm or cold compress by using a clean cloth or cotton swab. Use only boiled or purified water to wet the cloth and place this on the closed eye. A warm compress typically helps to reduce discomfort, while a cold compress works well to reduce itchiness and inflammation **(Marilyn and David, 2007).**

Eye diseases and infections are fairly easily prevented. Just by taking a few precautions, you can avoid many bothersome eye conditions: wash your hands before and after touching your eyes or face. If you have allergies, try your best to avoid allergens and keep an allergy-free living environment. Avoid foods that trigger reactions. Do not share contact lens equipment, containers or solutions and ensure that you keep the lenses sterile. Never use saliva in place of contact solution. Don't share towels, pillows or washcloths with others, especially if they have an eye infection or other viral and bacterial condition such as cold sores. Changes pillowcases and wash towels and bedding frequently. Use immune system boosters to boost your immune system to help prevent infection as well as to encourage faster healing **(Sheikh et al., 2008).**

C) Malaria:

WHO (2012) is defined malaria as it is a disease that is transmitted by the bite of a particular kind of mosquito. There are four main strains of malaria. The most serious of these is the **falciparum**. This form can be fatal. The other three forms, **vivax, ovale** and **malariae** are usually less serious, but still need to be prevented and treated promptly. 1.2 million people die every year world wide due to malaria resulting from inadequate sanitation facilities.

Symptom of malaria can be varied. Usually the symptoms include high fever, chills, headache, feeling unwell, muscle aches and cramps. Treatment of malaria there are 5 types of anti malarial medication that are stocked at travel clinic matraville. It is important to note that none of the anti malarial drugs are 100% effective in preventing malaria. These drugs are chloroquin, malarone, doxycycline, proguanil and lariam **(WHO, 2012).**

Prevention of malaria are avoid mosquito in general by avoid accumulation of waste that the mosquito are spread in this waste , care of house cleaning and use of an insect repellant containing Diethyl Emeta Tolumide (DEET), such as RID **(WHO, 2012).**

d) Parasitic disease:

A parasitic disease is an infectious disease caused or transmitted by a parasite. Many parasites don't cause diseases. Parasitic diseases can affect practically all living organisms, including plants and mammals. The study of parasitic diseases is called parasitology. Some parasites like toxoplasma gondii and plasmodium spp. can cause disease directly, but other organisms can cause disease by the toxins that they produce. Although organisms such as bacteria function as parasites, the usage of term "parasitic disease" is usually more restricted. The three main types of organisms causing these conditions are protozoa (causing protozoan infection), helminthes (helminthiasis) and ectoparasites. Protozoa and helminthes are usually endoparasites (usually living inside the body of the host),

42

while ectoparasites usually live on the surface of the host. Occasionally the definition of "parasitic disease" is restricted to diseases due to endoparasites **(WHO, 2010).**

Mammals can get parasites from contaminated food or water, bug bites, or sexual contact. Ingestion of contaminated water can produce Giardia infections. Parasites normally enter the body through the skin or mouth. Close contact with pets can lead to parasite infestation as dogs and cats are host to many parasites. Other risks that can lead people to get parasites are walking barefeet, inadequate disposal of faeces, lack of hygiene, close contact with someone who carries specific parasites and eating undercooked or exotic foods **(CDC, 2010).**

Symptoms of parasites may not always be obvious. Actually, such symptoms may mimic anemia or a hormone deficiency. Some of the symptoms caused by several worm infestation can include itching affecting the anus or the vaginal area, abdominal pain, weight loss, increased appetite, bowel obstructions, diarrhea and vomiting eventually leading to dehydration, sleeping problems, worms present in the vomit or stools, anemia, aching muscles or joints, general malaise, allergies, fatigue, nervousness. Symptoms may also be confused with pneumonia or food poisoning **(CDC, 2010).**

The effects caused by parasitic diseases range from mild discomfort to death. The nematode parasites necator Americans and ancylostoma duodenal cause human hookworm infection which leads to anemia and protein malnutrition. This infection affects approximately 740 million people in the developing countries, including children and adults, of the tropics specifically in poor rural areas located in sub-Saharan Africa, Latin America, South-East Asia and China. Chronic hookworm in children leads to impaired physical and intellectual development, school performance and attendance are reduced. Pregnant women affected by a hookworm infection can also develop anemia which results in negative outcomes both for the mother and the infant. Some of them are: low birth weight, impaired milk production, as well as increased risk of death for the mother and the baby **(CDC, 2010).**

Albendazole and mebendazole have been the treatments administered to entire populations to control hookworm infection. However, it is a costly option and both children and adults become reinfected within a few months after deparasitation occurs raising concerns because the treatment has to repeatedly be administered and drug resistance may occur **(Keen, 2013).**

Another medication administered to kill worm infections has been pyrantel pamoate. For some parasitic diseases there is no treatment and in the case of serious symptoms, medication intended to kill the parasite is administered, while in other cases, symptom relief options are used **(Hyman et al., 2013).**

e) Skin diseases:

An inflammation of the skin is an infection of the skin. Infection of the skin is distinguished from dermatitis which s inflammation of the skin, but a skin infection can result in skin inflammation. Skin inflammation due to skin infection is called infective dermatitis **(David et al., 2009)**.

Causes of skin diseases:

1. Bacterial:

David et al (2009) mentioned the bacterial cause of skin disease as the following:

- Impetigo is a highly contagious bacterial skin infection most common among pre-school children. It is primarily caused by Staphylococcus aureus, and sometimes by Streptococcus pyogenes.
- Erysipelas is an acute streptococcus bacterial infection of the deep epidermis with lymphatic spread.
- Cellulites is a diffuse inflammation of connective tissue with severe inflammation of dermal and subcutaneous layers of the skin.

Cellulites can be caused by normal skin flora or by exogenous bacteria and often occurs where the skin has previously been broken: cracks in the skin, cuts, blisters, burns, insect bites, surgical wounds; intravenous drug injection or sites of intravenous catheter insertion. Skin on the face or lower legs is most commonly affected by this infection though cellulites can occur on any part of the body.

2. Fungal:

Fungal skin infections may present as either a superficial or deep infection of the skin, hair and or nails. They affect about one billion people globally **(Vos, 2012)**.

3. Parasitic infestations, stings, and bites:

Parasitic infestations, stings and bites in humans are caused by several groups of organisms belonging to the following phyla: annelida, arthropods, bryozoa, chordate, cindaria, cyanobacteria, echinodermata, nemathelminthes, platyhelminthes and protozoa **(Diaz, 2010).**

4. Viral:

Viruses-related cutaneous conditions are caused by two main groups of viruses-DNA and RNA types-both of which are obligatory intracellular parasites **(Lebwohl et al, 2010).**

Maseleno and Hasan (2012) mentioned precaution should be taken to prevent skin infection:

- Avoid contact with person affected by one of skin diseases.
- Hand washing before and after eat.
- Hand washing after contact with any person affected with skin diseases.
- Don't use patient personal equipment as toile or billow.
- When you have any symptom of skin diseases you should go to physician and take treatment as prescribed.
- Avoid touch patient equipment.
- Isolate patient if the patient status are chronic.

f) Poisoning:

Most poisoning accidents involve swallowing of drugs, household products and food poisoning, insecticides...etc. Some poisoning agents can cause breathing difficulties, seek medical attention immediately **(Shannon, 2003)**.

Sings and symptoms of poisoning are generally, food poisoning causes some combination of nausea, vomiting, and diarrhea that may or may not be bloody, sometimes with other symptoms. After eating tainted food, abdominal cramps, diarrhea, and vomiting, can start as early as one hour in the case of staph and as late as 10 days in the case of campylobacter. It may take even longer to develop symptoms from parasite infections such as Giardia. Symptoms can last from one day up to a couple of months or longer, depending on the type of infection. Vomiting, diarrhea, sweating, dizziness, tearing in the eyes, excessive salivation, mental confusion, and stomach pain may be symptoms of chemical or toxin food poisoning such as that from poisonous mushrooms. Partial loss of speech or vision, muscle weakness, difficulty swallowing, dry mouth, muscle paralysis from the head down through the body, and vomiting may indicate botulism, a severe but very rare type of bacterial food poisoning **(URAC, 2013)**.

Nies and McEwen (2012) mentioned the treatment of poisoning as the following : Some people who have swallowed a poisonous substance or have overdosed on medication will be admitted to hospital for examination.

Possible treatments that can be used to treat poisoning include:

- **Activated charcoal** - healthcare professionals sometimes use activated charcoal (charcoal that has been treated so that it is pure carbon) to treat someone who has been poisoned. The charcoal binds to the poison and stops it from being further absorbed into the blood.
- **Antidotes** - these are substances that either prevent the poison from working or reverse the effects of the poison.
- **Sedatives** - these may be given if the person is agitated.
- **A ventilator (breathing machine)** - this may be used if the person stops breathing.
- **Anti-epileptic medicine** - this may be used if the person has seizures .

Prevention, keep medicine and chemicals out of sight and reach of children, preferably in an isolated, locked cabinet, always store chemicals in their original containers with appropriate labels, never tell children drugs are "sweets" as this may give a wrong idea to children. Ensure toys and dining utensils bought meet the international standard e.g. coloring materials being non-toxic **(Shannon, 2003).**

g) Scorpion bite:

Scorpions are long and the body ends in a narrow, tail-like structure with a curved stinger. The stinger delivers neurotoxic venom to paralyze larger prey. The front pair of a scorpion's appendages are enlarged and equipped with pincers, similar to those of a crab or cray fish, which are used to hold prey for stinging and

48

feeding. Scorpions also sting in self-defense. Scorpions hold their tails curled upward over their backs. To sting, the tail and tinger are thrust back and downward, injecting toxin through the stinger into the victim. Scorpions search at night for insects and spiders to eat, and to find mates. Indoor problems with scorpions are most frequently encountered where homes or other buildings are located close to outcroppings of rock layers. In their nightly wanderings, scorpions readily enter man-made structures. Crevices around foundations and beneath doors may even be attractive to them as places to hide. Scorpions mostly inhabit in dry and warm areas **(Zurek, 2005).**

Bawaskar and Bawaskar (2007) mentioned clinical effects of the envenomation as the following:- clinical effects depends upon the species of scorpion and lethality and dose of venom injected at the time of sting. Severe effects are seen in first victim than envenomed by same scorpion to subsequent victim. Severity of envenoming is related to age, size of scorpion and the season of the sting and time lapsed between sting and hospitalization. Children who have been stung by a bark scorpion might experience:

• Pain, which can be intense, numbness and tingling in the area around the sting, but little or no swelling
• Muscle twitching or thrashing
• Unusual head, neck and eye movements
• Drooling
• Sweating
• Restlessness or excitability and sometimes inconsolable crying.

Adults are more likely to experience:

- Rapid breathing
- High blood pressure
- Increased heart rate
- Muscle twitching
- Weakness.

Charlotte (2006) mentioned scorpions bite treatment :

1. Wash the sting with soap and water and remove all jewelry.
2. Apply cool compresses.
3. Acetaminophen (Tylenol) 1-2 tablets every 4 hours may be given to relieve pain. Avoid aspirin and ibuprofen.
4. Antibiotics are not helpful.
5. Do not cut into the wound or apply suction.

To prevent spread of scorpions in the house should don't leave shoes, boots, clothing items or wet towels outdoors where scorpions can hide. Shake towels around the swimming pool and shake all clothing and shoes before putting them on. Wear gloves when working in the yard. Wear shoes outdoors, especially during the evening hours. A portable black light Ultra violet light may be used to survey for scorpions in and around the home. Scorpions glow brightly under black light and are therefore easily found and removed. Scorpions can enter buildings through openings around plumbing fixtures and loose-fitting doors and windows as well as cracks in foundations and walls. Outdoor lights attract insects and thus the scorpions that feed on insects. Yellow outdoor lighting is less attractive to insects and is recommended in areas where scorpions are prevalent. The first strategy for control is to modify the area surrounding a house, because scorpions are difficult to control with insecticides. Use the following checklist to protect the house:

• Clean the yard by removing all trash, logs, boards, stones, bricks, and other objects from around the foundation of the home.

• Prune overhanging tree branches away from the house, because they can provide a path to the roof for scorpions.

• Don't store firewood inside the house; bring in only wood to be directly placed on the fire, and check for scorpions before bringing the wood inside.

• Install weather stripping around loose-fitting doors and windows.

• Caulk around roof eaves, pipes, and any other cracks that allow entrance into the home.

• Make sure window screens fit tightly in the window frame, and keep the screens in good repair. screens in good repair **(Mallis et al., 2004).**

h) Snakes bites:

Snakes bites is an injury caused by a bite from a snake, often resulting in puncture wounds inflicted by the animal's fangs and sometimes resulting in envenomation. Although the majority of snake species are non-venomous and typically kill their prey with constriction rather than venom, venomous snakes can be found on every continent except Antarctica **(Kasturiratne et al., 2008)**. Snakes often bite their prey as a method of hunting, but also for defensive purposes against predators. Since the physical appearance of snakes may differ, there is often no practical way to identify a species and professional medical attention should be sought (**White and Julian, 2006).**

Snake bite's symptoms depend on numerous factors, including the species of snake, the area of the body bitten, the amount of venom injected and the health conditions of the person. Feelings of terror and panic are common after snakebite and can produce a characteristic set of symptoms mediated by the autonomic nervous system, such as a racing heart and nausea. Bites from non-venomous snakes can also cause injury, often due to lacerations caused by the snake's teeth or from a resulting infection. A bite may also trigger an anaphylactic reaction, which is potentially fatal **(Gold et al., 2002).**

The most common symptoms of all snakebites are overwhelming fear, panic, and emotional instability, which may cause symptoms such as nausea and vomiting, vertigo, fainting, tachycardia and cold, clammy skin. Television, literature and folklore are in part responsible for the hype surrounding snakebites and people may have unwarranted thoughts of imminent death **(Kitchens and Van Mierop, 2000).**

Valenta and Jiri (2010) mentioned that snakebite first aid recommendations vary, in part because different snakes have different types of venom. Some have little local effect, but life-threatening systemic effects, in which case containing the venom in the region of the bite by pressure immobilization is desirable. Other venoms instigate localized tissue damage around the bitten area, and immobilization may increase the severity of the damage in this area, but also reduce the total area affected; whether this trade-off is desirable remains a point of controversy. Because snakes vary from one country to another, first aid methods also vary.

Valenta and Jiri (2010) mentioned first aid guidelines agree on the following:

1. Protect the person and others from further bites. While identifying the species is desirable in certain regions, risking further bites or delaying proper medical treatment by attempting to capture or kill the snake is not recommended.

2. Keep the person calm. Acute stress reaction increases blood flow and endangers the person. Panic is infectious and compromises judgment.

3. Call for help to arrange for transport to the nearest hospital emergency room, where anti venom for snakes common to the area will often be available.

4. Make sure to keep the bitten limb in a functional position and below the person's heart level so as to minimize blood returning to the heart and other organs of the body.

5. Do not give the person anything to eat or drink. This is especially important with consumable alcohol, a known vasodilator which will speed up the absorption of venom. Do not administer stimulants or pain medications, unless specifically directed to do so by a physician.

6. Remove any items or clothing which may constrict the bitten limb if it swells (rings, bracelets, watches, footwear, etc.)

7. Keep the person as still as possible.

8. Get to Hospital Immediately. Traditional remedies have no proven benefit in treating snakebite.

9. Do not incise the bitten site.

Prevention of snake bites according to (Organizational Health, 2013):

As always, prevention is better than cure.

• Take care when clearing vegetation, raking dry leaves in your garden. Supervise kids in the outdoors, especially in a green neighborhood.

• Use torch/flashlight at night and keep wearing those shoes. Check shoes before wearing them.

• Watch your step and see before you sit!

• Keep the backyard free of junk and make sure the solid waste is managed properly.

• If see a snake, do nothing, Let it go. Do not try to pick it up or kill it. If a snake has entered the premises, call professional snake rescuers.

• Minimize the food sources for snakes by removing anything that may attract rodents or frogs.

• Reduce rubbish/materials where a snake could shelter.

• During high risk times or after holiday breaks, remind staff and students of the increased risk of the presence of snakes.

• Wear gloves and boots when moving stored materials and rubbish - they will give some protection.

• An increased awareness of snakes is the best protection. The snake will not be looking for you, so be alert and on the lookout for snakes.

9- The role of the community health nurse in prevention of diseases caused by waste accumulation:

CHN can encourage the positive action described by educating the public, nurse can promote greater sensitivity among citizen to the problems of accumulating waste with its potential health hazards. Public cooperation with organized refuse collection will require a considerable effort by community worker. Nurse encourage client to buy products that can be recycled and discourage use of non recyclable items. CHN must sharing information with people during home visits and make family and home assessment **(Allender et al., 2010).** The primary responsibilities of the CHN are advocacy and education of the client in the home, at work and in the community. Primary prevention is to focus of the educating people about safe solid wastes disposal methods. Nurse make intervention to help in minimizing the potential for illness transmission from insect and rodents that can come in contact with infectious agents and spread disease **(Smith and Maurer, 2000).**

Nurses are important to environmental health because they play key roles in protecting the health of all people, are in direct contact with patients, families and communities from many cultural and socioeconomic backgrounds and have the credibility and access that enables them to provide scientifically sound information about environmental issues and toxic exposures **(Spradely and Allender, 2008).**

The role of CHN in prevention and control of environmental health hazards include primary, secondary and tertiary prevention. **Primary level of prevention** relates to activities direct at preventing a problem before it occurs. Primary prevention is involved in both health promotion and disease prevention. Health promotion activities enhance resources directed at improving well-being. Disease prevention begins with recognition of a health risk, a disease or environmental hazards and is followed by measures to protect as many people as possible from harmful consequences of that risk. In addition to, development of a disease is avoided. Most population based health promotion activities are primary preventive measures e.g. hand Washing, immunization, personal hygiene, positive health habits **(Killer et al., 2004).**

Secondary level of prevention, strategies are aimed at early diagnosis, early treatment interventions and attempts to limit disability through assess homes for environmental hazards. Preventive activities are aimed at early disease detection thereby increasing opportunities for interventions to prevent progression of the diseases and emergency of symptoms e.g. early treatment of diseases **(Nies and McEwen, 2012).**

Tertiary level of prevention, CHN are encourage clean up of toxic waste sites and removable of waste hazards. Provide appropriate nursing care at home or work sites for persons with chronic disease and injury. Reduces the negative impact of an already established disease by restoring function and reducing disease related complications e.g. rehabilitative measures. These are based on five levels of control:

a. Health Promotion

b. Specific disease prevention

c. Early diagnosis and treatment

d. Limitation of disabilities

e. Rehabilitation **(Keller et al., 2004).**

References:

1. **Abul, S. (2010):** Environmental and health impact of solid waste disposal at management dumpsite in Manzini: Swaziland. Journal of sustainable development in Africa 12(7) p.70.

2. **Agwu, M. (2012):** Issues and challenges of solid waste management practices in Port-Harcourt city, Nigeria-behavioral perspective. Am. J. Soc. Mgmt. Sci, 3(2) p. 83-92.

3. **Allender, J.A. Rector ,C. and Warner, K.D. (2010):** Public Health Essentials for Community Health Nursing, Community Health Nursing, Promoting and protecting the publics Health. Philadelphia. Chapter(9),7th ed New York, p.261.

4. **Azikiwe, N. Ifeoma, M. Ugochukwu, O. and Nkiru, E. (2013):** Public Health Implication of Household Solid Waste Management in Awka south east Nigeria. Accessed on line http: // archive. ispub. com: 80/ journal/ the-internet- journal –of- public –health/ volume-1- number-1/ public-health- implication- of-household-solid-waste-management-in-Awka-south-east- Nigeria-html.

5. **Bawaskar, HS. and Bawaskar, PH. (2007):** Consecutive sting by red scorpion evokes severe cardiovascular manifestations in the first, but not in the second victim: a clinical observation. J Trop Med Hyg; 9(4) p 231-33.

6. **Caroline, M. (2008):** Inflammation of the eye. NetDoctor.co.uk is a trademark PDF. P.132-143.

7. **CDC, Centers for Diseases Control and Prevention, (2010):"** Parasitic diseases causes and symptom " Retrieved 2010. Jan; 12(1) p.11-15.

8. **Charlotte, G. (2006):** First aids emergencies. scorpions stings treatment. for more information (http://www.emedicinehealth.com/script/ main/art.asp? articlekey=59026). p.15-20.

9. **David, J. DiCaudo; Dirk Elston, MD. Dirk, M. Elston; Tammie Ferringer; Christine, J. Ko; Christine Ko MD; Steven Peckham and Whitney, A. (2009):** Dermatopathology. Philadelphia: Saunders. ISBN 0- 7020-3023-6.

10. **Diaz, J. (2010):** "Mite-transmitted dermatoses and infectious diseases in returning travelers". J Travel Med 17 (1): p. 21–31.

11. **Duane, J. (1998):** Resurgent Vector-Borne Diseases as a Global Health Problem, Emerging infectious Diseases, vol. 5(4): p.3-5.

12. **Ekemini, I. (2012):** Problems and prospects of waste disposal in Port-Harcourt metropolis. Master thesis. p.66.

13. **EL-zanaty,F, and Way, A. (2009):** Egypt Demographic and Health Survey. Cairo, Egypt: Ministry of Health, Unicef, USAID and El-Zanaty and Associates. Sanitation facilities and waste disposal, p 15, 21-22.

14. **Fischer, C. and Crowe, M. (2000):** Household and municipal waste. Comparability of Data in European

Environment Agency member countries. Copenhagen: European Environment Agency. Envi. Health.(6)2. pp. 143-150.

15. **Goddard, J. (2000):** Infectious Diseases and Arthropods in Totwa, P.120- 130.

16. **Gold, B. Richard C. Dart, B. and Robert, A. (2002):** "Bites of venomous snakes". The New England Journal of Medicine, 347 (5): pp. 347–56.

17. **Gonzalez-Reuiz, A. Haque, R. and Rehman, T. (2009):** Diagnosis of amebic dysentery by detection of Entamobia histolytica fecal antigen by an invasive strain-specific, monoclonal antibody-based enzyme-linked immunosorbent assay. J Clin Microbiol, 32(4): pp. 964-70.

18. **Greenberg, H. and Estes, M. (2009):** "Rotaviruses: from pathogenesis to vaccination". Gastroenterology, 136 (6): pp. 1939-51.

19. **Hassan, A. Abd Elrahman, N. and Syed, SH. (2008):** The level of environmental knowledge, awareness, attitudes and practice among university Kebangsaan Malaysia. pp. 20-23.

20. **Hyman, P. Atterbury, R. and Barrow, P. (2013)**: "Fleas and smaller fleas: Virotherapy for parasite infections". Trends in Microbiology, 21 (5): pp. 215–220.

21. **Jamias, S. and Tatlonghari, R. (2010):** Village level knowledge, attitudes and practices on solid waste management in Sta. Rosa city, Laguna, Philippines. J. Env. Science and

management, 13(1): pp. 35-51.

22. **Jonton, A. (2006):** Household Participation in Domestic Waste Disposal and Recycling in the Tshwane Metropolitan Area : An Environmental Education Perspective. pp. 12-16.

23. **Kaewsawang, S. (2002):** An evaluation of knowledge attitude and behavior of household and commercial sectors to solid waste select in Salaya municipality, Nakhornpathom province. Master Sc thesis in appropriate technology for resource development. Faculty of Graduate studies. Mahidol university. p. 75.

24. **Kasturiratne, A. Wickremasinghe, A. de Silva, N. and Gunawardena, N. (2008):** "The Global Burden of snakebite: A literature Analysis and Modelling Based on Regional Estimates of Envenoming and Deaths". In Winkel, Ken. PloS Medicine, 5 (11): p. 218.

25. **Keen, E. (2013):** "Beyond phage therapy: Virotherapy of protozoal diseases". Future Microbiology, 8 (7): pp. 821–823.

26. **Keller, L. Strohschein, S. Lia-Hoagberg, B. and Schaffer, M. (2004):** Population- based public health intervention: practice based and evidence supported. public health nursing. 21(5): pp. 453-468.

27. **Khalaf, F. (2012):** Knowledge and attitude of Assiut University Dorms students about consanguinity marriage. Subjects and Methods. Faculty of Nursing, Assiut University. p.59.

28. **Kitchens, A. and Van Mierop, D. (2000):** "Envenomation by the Eastern coral snake (Micrurus fulvius fulvius). A study of 39 victims". JAMA, 258 (12): pp. 1615–18.

29. **Ladu, J. Osman, M. and Lu, X. (2012):** Solid waste management and its environmental impacts on human health in Juba town – south Sudan. Scholarly Journals of Biotechnology, 1(2): p. 34-35.

30. **Language, P. and Van Blerk, J. (2000):** Recycling and ferrochrome furnace Bagfilter Dust out samancor chrome- A Success story. Clear Air Journal. vol, 10 (5): p. 15-22.

31. **Lebwohl, M. Rosen, T. and Stockfleth, E. (2010):** "The role of human papillomavirus in common skin conditions: current viewpoints and therapeutic options". Cutis 86 (5): p. 11-12.

32. **Long, E. and Kehinde, M. (2005):** Investigation of potential ground water impacts at an unlined waste disposal site in Agege, Lagos, Nigeria. pro 3rd Faculty of Engineering International Conference, University of Lagos, Nigeria, p 21-29.

33. **Longe, E. and Williams, A. (2006):** A preliminary study of medical Waste management in Lagos metropolis, Nigeria, Iranian J. Env. Health sci. Eng. 3(2): pp. 133-9.

34. **Longe, O. Longe, E. and Ukpebor, E. (2009):** People's Perception on Household Solid Waste Management in Ojo Local Government Area in Nigeria. Iran. J. Environ. Health sci. Eng. 6 (3): pp. 212-14.

35.   **Mahmoud, T. (2010):** Assessment of home environment and its relation to children's health as a basis to design an educational program for their mothers in rural areas in Assiut governorate. Doctor thesis. Review of literature. p.46.

36.   **Mallis, A. Moreland, S. and Hedges, A. (2004):** The Mallis Handbook of Pest Control. 9th ed. Richfield, OH: GIE Media Inc. p.50.

37.   **Makmattayan, R. (2003):** Factors related to solid waste sorting behavior among housewives in Bang sue district, Bangkok . Master thesis in environmental education. Faculty of Graduate studies, Mahidol University. p.80.

38.   **Marilyn, J. and David, M. (2007):** Nursing care of infants and children. 8th Edition. Mosby. Pp 1366-69.

39.   **Marshall, T. (2005):** Inflammation of the eye, posted: Fri Oct 7th, 00:59. Journal of Medical Health. 5(3). p.15-20.

40.   **Maseleno, A. and Hasan, M. (2012):** "Skin Diseases Expert System using Dempster-Shafer Theory". International Journal of Intelligent Systems and Applications, 4 (5): p. 38–44.

41.   **Mengistie, N. and Baraki, B. (2010):** Community based assessment on household management of waste and hygiene practice in Kersa Wored, Eastern Ethiopia, Ethiop. J. Health Der. 2010; 24(2): p. 105.

42.   **Miller, G. (2002):** Living in the Environment. principles, connection and solution wads worth Group Brook/ Cole, 2nd

Edition. Philadelphia. p.4-7.

43. **Min, M. (2009):** Environmental health and sanitation conditions among Myanmar migrant communities in Samut Sakorn province Thailand. Proceeding of the 41st APACPH conference, Taiwan. p. 90.

44. **Ministry of Public Health and Sanitation. (2011):** Fact sheet about sanitation and hygiene promotion. p. 3-5.

45. **Mitchell, D. (2002):** "Astrovirus gastroenteritis". The Pediatric Infectious Disease Journal, 21 (11): pp. 1067-1069.

46. **Moghadam, M. and Ehrampoush, M. (2005):** Survey of knowledge, attitude and practice of Yazd university of medical sciences student about solid wastes disposal and recycling. Iranian J Env Health Sci Eng, vol (2) No (2), pp. 26-30.

47. **Mohammed, J. (2010):** Assessment of nursing intervention for nurse working with elderly burned patients as a basis for designing of an educational program for them in Assiut city. Unpublished Thesis Doctor, Faculty of Nursing, Assiut University. p.50.

48. **Mohee, R. (2001):** Waste management opportunities for rural Communities Composting as an effective waste management strategy for farm households and others. Ministry of Local Government, Port Louis. Mauritius. p. 90-93.

49. **Naing, Y. (2009):** Factors influencing the practice of household waste management among Myanmar migrant in muang

district, Ranong province, Thailand. p.4-5, 73-7.

50. **Navaneethan, U. and Giannella, R. (2008):** Mechanisms of infectious diarrhea. Nature clinical practice. Gastroenterology & hepatology, 5(11): pp. 637-47.

51. **Nies, M. and McEwen, M. (2012):** Factors that influence the Health of the Community – Community /Public Health Nursing, Promoting the Health of Population, chap(3),5th ed, New York. Pp. 248-50, 1455-1457.

52. **Nour Eldeen, M. (2011):** Environmental Health awareness Scale : A proposed Model for Egypt As a Developing Country. Pp. 56-61.

53. **NRDC. (2006):** Facts About Pollution from Livestock Farms, Natural   Resources Defense Council. p.40.

54. **Okechukwu, O. Okechukwu, A. Noye-Nortey, H. and Owusu Agyei. (2012):** Health perception of indiscriminate waste disposal- Achanaian case study. Journal of medicine and medical sciences vol. 3(3) p. 151.

55. **Organizational Health. (2013):** Health and Safety Fact Sheet preventing   and   managing   snakes   bites. http://www.snake/snakesbite preventing/PDF/fact sheet. PDF. p. 33.

56. **Owaduge, S. (2010):** Solid Waste Management in Lokoja metropolis.   Accessed   online. (http://www.greatestcities.com/users/owagde).

57. **Padma, L. Tabunakawai, M. and Singh, S. (2006):** Economics of rural waste management in the Rewa Province and development of rural solid waste management policy for fiji. Master thesis. P.7.

58. **Pheby, D. Grey, M. Giusti, L. and Saffron, L. (2002):** Waste Management and Public Health: The State of the Evidence. Bristol: South West Public Health Observatory. p. 20.

59. **Prescott, N. Palaki, A. Tongia, S. and Niu, L. (2004):** Household survey and waste characterization for Nukuhetulu, Tonga. pp. 27-29.

60. **Sachs, J. and Malaney, P. (2002):** The economic and social burden of malaria nature 415(2) : pp. 680-685.

61. **Schiller, L. (2007):** "Management of diarrhea in clinical practice: strategies for primary care physicians". Rev Gastroenterol Disord 7 Suppl 3 : p. 27-38.

62. **Shannon, M. (2003):** Primary care ingestion of toxic substances by children, N England Journal of Medical Science, 342 (3) : pp. 186-191.

63. **Sheikh, A. Hurwitz, B. and Cave, J. (2008):** Antibiotics for acute bacterial conjunctivitis. Cochrane Library. Issue 3,8 (1): p. 3-21.

64. **Smith, C. and Maurer, F. (2000):** Community Health Nursing Theory and Practice, Environmental Issues: At Home, at Work and in the Community, chapter (24), 4th ed, London. P.665.

65. **Solano, M. Iriarte, F. Ciria, P. and Negro, M. (2001):** Performance characteristics of three aeration systems in the composting of sheep Manure and straw. J of Agr Eng Res. 79(3): pp. 317–329.

66. **Spardley, B. and Allender, J. (2008):** Community Health Nursing Concept and Practice, Environmental Health and Safety, chapter (6), 7th ed, New York. pp. 131-133.

67. **Tadesse, T. (2004):** Solid waste management. Introduction to solid waste management. p.7-9.

68. **United Nation. (2000):** Fact sheet about solid waste disposal , (http://www.un-org/waste/waste/disposal/pdf/factsheet.PDF).

69. **United State Environment Protection Agency. (2006):** Informal Solid Waste management. (http://www.unep.org?PDF/Kenyawastemngnt sector/ Sector/chapter/PDF).

70. **United Nations Environment Programme. (2000):** International Source Book Environmentally Sound Technologies (ESTs) for Municipal Solid Waste Management(MSWM). p.90-8.

71. **UNEP (United Nation Environmental Programme). (2002):** Environmental Data Report 2000/2001. A-Report for global Environmental Monitoring System. Brazil. Black well, Oxford. UK. pp. 805-18.

72. **URAC . (2013):** Food poisoning health center. Food poisoning sings and symptoms. p.65.

73. **Valenta, A. and Jiri, D. (2010):** Venomous Snakes: Envenoming, Therapy (2nd ed.). Hauppauge, New York: Nova Science Publishers. ISBN 978-1-60876-618-5.

74. **Van Beukering, P. Sehker, M. Gerlagh, R. and Kumar, V. (2005):** Analyzing Urban Solid Waste in Developing Countries: A perspective on Bangalore, India. International Institute for Environmental and Development (IIEP). Working paper No. 24 CREED Working Paper Series. Amsterdam.

75. **Vos, T. (2012):** "Years lived with disability (YLDs) for 1160 sequelae of 289 diseases and injuries 1990-2010: a systematic analysis for the Global Burden of Disease Study 2010.". Lancet, 380 (9859): 2163–96.

76. **Wallinga, D. (2004):** Concentrated Animal Feeding Operations: Health Risks from Air Pollution. Minneapolis, Institute for Agriculture and Trade Policy, Food and Health Program. p.80.

77. **Wangen, S. (2006):** The irritable Bowel Syndrome Solution.; Innate Health Publishing P:113. ISBN 968-0-9768537-8-7. Excerpted with the author's permission at http://www.IBSTTreatmentCenter.com.

78. **Water Sanitation and Hygiene-Alek base (2012):** Knowledge, attitude and practice survey report Gogrial west county, Warrap state. South Sudan, solid waste management. p.10.

79. **White, A. and Julian, E. (2006):** Snakebite and spider bite: Management Guidelines. Adelaide: Department of Health, Government of South Australia. pp. 1–71.

80. **World Health Organization. (2000):** Department of Communicable Disease Surveillance and Response See http://www.who.int/emc for more information.

81. **World Health Organization. (2005):** the effects of air pollution in a number of areas. p.59.

82. **World Health Organization. (2007):** fact sheet on cholera. Last up-date September 2007 http://www.who.int/mediacentre/factsheets/fs107/en/.

83. **World Health Organization. (2010):** "Intestinal protozoal Diseases: medicines pediatrics: General Medicine" . p.54.

84. **World Health Organization. (2012):** Travel Clinic Matraville a division of Matraville medical complex. malaria disease information sheets. http://www.who.int/vaccination.com. p.60.

85. **Zayani, A. and Riad M. (2010):** Solid waste management overview and current status in Egypt. p.13.

86. **Zurek, L. (2005):** Pests that affect human health. spiders and scorpions effect on health of human. p.4.

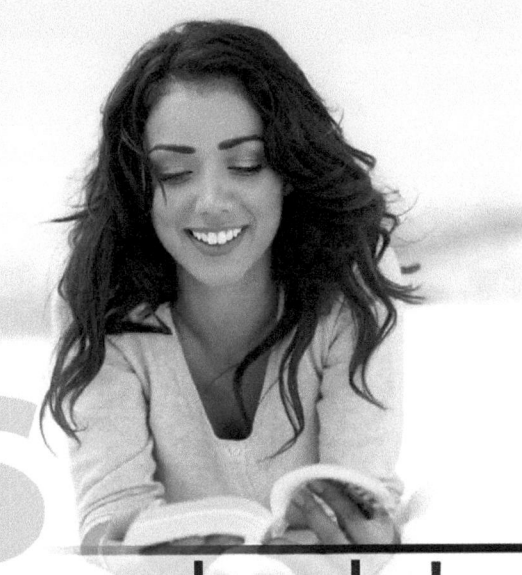
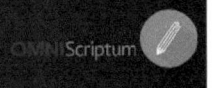

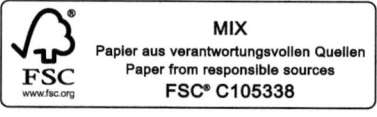